CW00524787

The Complete Copycat Recipes

Easy and Tasty Recipes for 365 Days. Start Making the Most Famous Restaurant Dishes at Home. Steakhouses, Chipotle, Fast Food, Cracker Barrel and much more.

JORDAN BERGSTROM

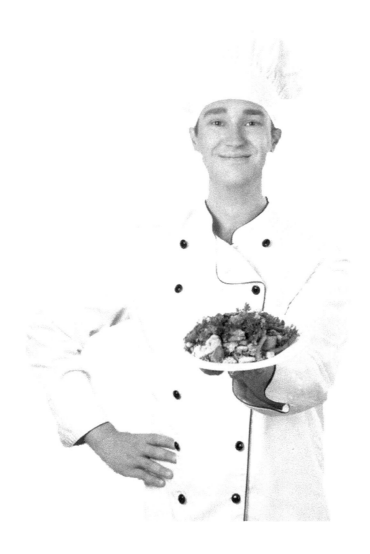

TABLE OF CONTENTS

INTRODUCTION

Only a few things are more satisfying than sinking your teeth into a home-cooked meal. From Meatloaf to Pound Cake, this book covers how to make every dish your family craves. Go old school with these classics or indulge with newer entrees.

What is Copycat Recipe?

A copycat recipe is a recipe that attempts to recreate the taste of another restaurant's meal through substitution of ingredients and cooking processes. Regular home cooking relies on experiential knowledge that could be difficult to convey in written form.

Two ways how Copycat Recipe contributes to the rhetoric in the industry:

1. Economically: It is a gateway to imitate and create products that don't require much financial investment, and thus save families money. Copycat recipes are also commonly adapted for personal reasons, such as religious dietary considerations.
2. Socially: The book introduces people to new ingredients and recipes, as well as the concepts of variety and experimentation with food.

Benefits of Dining in Your Home Rather than Going Out

1. Save money. Restaurant prices are ridiculously high, and there is no reason why you should pay above the market price for a meal.
2. Stay healthier. Restaurant-prepared meals are often higher in fat, salt and sugar than what you would consume in your home or make at home to eat in restaurants.
3. It's fun to cook. Many people resort to take-out (such as Subway) because it is easier than cooking at home. Cooking at home may look difficult, but it's actually a lot of fun if you have the right skills and resources.
4. It's cheaper to cook at home. Not only can you save money on ingredients, but there's no tip involved when you eat at home. There are also fewer dishes to wash and store later.
5. You're in control of what you eat. When eating out, it is easy to make poor food choices if you do not know what is in the food that you are consuming.

How Does Copycat Recipes Start?

Copycat Recipes was started by Cara Zuchora, who loves cooking and aspired to make her own food at home. The only problem was that she is a bad cook. She doesn't like eating prepared food and would rather cook everything for herself. From there, she decided to find ways to improve her cooking skills through literature research, and experimented with these tools in the kitchen.

Why Does Copycat Recipes Get Attention?

It helps families with special diets such as low-fat and vegetarian, as well as those who want to cut down the cost of their food bills. It can help preserve cultural recipes in a way that almost anyone can recreate them in their own kitchens.

This Copycat Recipe Book contains 100+ recipes that your family will surely love. So, let us start cooking. Enjoy!

BREAKFAST RECIPES

Cheesecake Pancakes

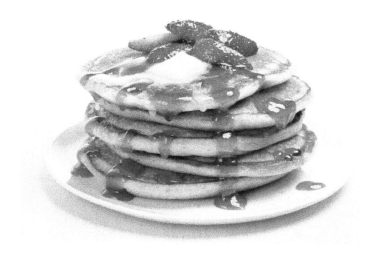

Preparation time: 10 minutes

Cooking Time: 6 minutes

Servings: 12

Ingredients:

Pancakes

- 1 package (8 oz) cream cheese
- 2 cups Original Bisquick™ mix
- ½ cup graham cracker crumbs
- ¼ cup sugar

- 1 cup milk

- 2 eggs

Strawberry Syrup

- 1 cup sliced fresh strawberries

- ½ cup strawberry syrup

Direction:

1. Cut cream cheese lengthwise into 4 pieces. Situate on ungreased cookie sheet; wrap and freeze 8 hours. Grease skillet with vegetable oil preheat griddle to 375°F.

2. Slice cream cheese into bite-size pieces; put aside. Mix Bisquick mix, graham cracker crumbs, sugar, milk and eggs with whisk or fork until blended. Stir in cream cheese.

3. For each pancake, Transfer slightly less than 1/3 cup batter onto hot griddle. Cook until edges are dry. Flip; cook other sides until golden brown.

4. Incorporate strawberries and syrup; top pancakes with strawberry mixture.

Nutrition: 132 Calories 5.3g Total fat 18.7g Carbohydrates

Starbucks Lemon Bread

Preparation Time: 15 minutes

Cooking Time: 50 minutes

Servings: 2

Ingredients:

- 1 ½ cups all-purpose flour
- 1/2 tsp. baking powder
- 1/4 tsp. baking soda
- 1/4 tsp. salt
- ½ cup unsalted butter softened
- 1 cup granulated sugar
- 3 big eggs
- ½ tsp. vanilla extract
- 1 tsp. lemon extract*
- zest of 1 large lemon
- 2 tbsp. lemon juice
- 1/3 cup buttermilk sour cream

Lemon Icing:

- 1 cup powdered sugar
- 1 tbsp. lemon juice
- 1 tbsp. cream or milk

Directions:

Lemon Loaf

1. Prep the oven to 350F degrees. Line and flour an 8 x 4-inch loaf pan with parchment paper.
2. Scourge flour, baking powder, baking soda & salt.
3. Blend butter and sugar until fluffy.
4. Mix in the eggs 1 simultaneously. Stir in the vanilla extract, optional lemon extract, lemon zest, and lemon juice.
5. Using mixer on low speed, stir in about 1/2 of the flour mixture then 1/2 of the buttermilk.
6. Do the process with the rest of the flour mixture and buttermilk.
7. Transfer batter into the greased pan then bake for 50-60 minutes. If after 37 minutes the top is browning too much, situate a piece of aluminum foil over top and continue baking.
8. Set aside the loaf fully before icing

Lemon Icing

1. Scourge powdered sugar, lemon juice, and cream/milk until smooth. Stir in more powdered sugar
2. Pull out the cooled loaf from the pan and drizzle or pour over top.

Nutrition: 477 Calories 20g Total fat 70.8g Carbohydrates

Barrel Cracker French Toast

Preparation Time: 1 minutes

Cooking Time: 5 minutes

Servings: 1

Ingredients:

- 8 slices Texas Toast (or Sourdough bread)
- 4 eggs
- 1 cup Milk
- 2 Tablespoons Sugar
- 4 teaspoons Vanilla extract
- 2 pinches of salt

Directions:

Incorporate eggs, milk, sugar, vanilla, and salt together in a large bowl.

Preheat griddle to 350F. Brush with butter/margarine.

1. Submerge the slice of bread in egg mixture for 30 seconds on each side.
2. Situate slices on griddle and cook for 4-5 minutes, or until golden brown.
3. Side with a pat of butter and your favorite syrup!

Nutrition: 1312 Calories 30.5g Total fat 191g Carbohydrates 54.1g Protein

Egg McMuffins

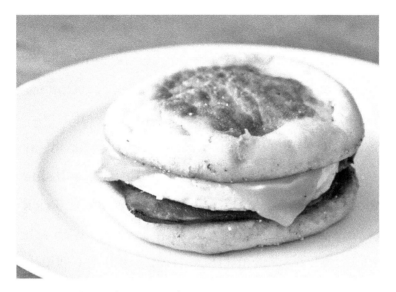

Preparation Time: 5 minutes

Cooking Time: 10 minutes

Servings: 2

Ingredients:

- 1 tablespoon unsalted butter
- 1 English muffin
- 1 slice high-quality Canadian bacon
- 1 large egg
- 1 slice Swiss, or Jack cheese

Direction:

1. Spread 1 tsp. butter on each halves of English muffin and situate halves in a 10-inch nonstick at medium heat.

Cook, then pressing gently to get good contact with pan for 4 minutes. Situate to a sheet of aluminum foil, split side up.

2. Cook remaining 1 teaspoon butter in the now-empty skillet and increase heat to medium-high. Fry bacon for 1 1/2 minutes. Situate bacon to lower muffin half.

3. Situate lid of a quart-sized, wide-mouthed Mason jar upside down in the now-empty skillet. Brush the inside with nonstick cooking spray and break egg into it. Prick the egg yolk with a fork to break it and season with salt and pepper. Stir in 3/4 cup (180ml) water into the skillet, cover, and cook until egg is set, about 2 minutes.

4. Using a thin spatula, situate Mason jar lid to a paper towel–lined plate. Take excess water out of the skillet and put it back to the stovetop with the heat off. Turn Mason jar lid over then gently remove it to release egg. Situate egg on top of bacon and garnish with cheese slice. Wrap with aluminum foil, and place it back to the now-empty skillet. Heat up in the skillet for 2 minutes with the heat off. Unwrap and serve immediately.

Nutrition: 96 Calories 12.8g Carbohydrates 5.3g Protein

Pumpkin Pancakes

Preparation Time: 10 minutes

Cooking Time: 10 minutes

Servings: 9

Ingredients:

- 1 ½ cups milk
- 1 cup pumpkin puree
- 1 egg
- 2 tablespoons vegetable oil
- 2 tablespoons vinegar
- 2 cups all-purpose flour
- 3 tablespoons brown sugar
- 2 teaspoons baking powder
- 1 teaspoon baking soda
- 1 teaspoon ground allspice
- 1 teaspoon ground cinnamon
- ½ teaspoon ground ginger
- ½ teaspoon salt

Directions:

1. Scourge milk, pumpkin, egg, oil and vinegar. Incorporate flour, brown sugar, baking powder, baking soda, allspice, cinnamon, ginger and salt in a separate bowl. Mix into the pumpkin mixture just enough to combine.

2. Preheat lightly oiled griddle or frying pan over medium high heat. Spoon batter onto the griddle, using approximately 1/4 cup for each pancake.

Nutrition: 134 Calories 5g Total fat 18g Carbohydrates

Frittata

Preparation Time: 5 minutes

Cooking Time: 20 minutes

Servings: 6

Ingredients:

- 6 large eggs
- ¼ cup heavy cream
- 1 tsp. kosher salt
- 4 slices thick-cut bacon
- 2 Yukon gold potatoes
- 1/4 tsp. freshly ground black pepper
- 2 cups baby spinach
- 2 cloves garlic
- 2 teaspoons fresh thyme leaves
- 1 cup shredded cheese

Directions:

1. Set to 400F and situate a rack in the middle of the oven.
2. Scourge eggs and cream together. Incorporate eggs, heavy cream, and 1/2 teaspoon salt together, put aside.
3. Situate bacon in a cold 10- to 12-inch nonstick oven safe frying pan, then turn the heat to medium-high. Fry bacon for 9 minutes. Take out bacon with a slotted spoon

to a paper towel-lined plate and scoop off all but 2 tablespoons of the fat.

4. Sauté the potatoes in bacon fat. Put the pan back to medium-heat, add the potatoes and sprinkle with the pepper and the remaining 1/2 teaspoon salt. Cook for 6 minutes.

5. Cook spinach with the garlic and thyme. Cook spinach into the pan with the garlic and thyme for 1 minute. Put bacon back to the pan and stir to evenly distribute.

6. Stir in cheese. Arrange vegetables into an even layer, flattening with a spatula. Drizzle cheese on top and let it just start to melt.

7. Transfer egg mixture into the skillet. Transfer egg mixture over the vegetables and cheese. Cook until you see the eggs at the edges of the pan beginning to set.

8. Bake for 9 minutes. Bake until the eggs are set.

9. Set aside. Serve

Nutrition: 324 Calories 2g Carbohydrates 19g Protein

Ragout

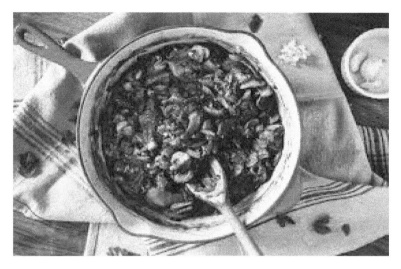

Preparation Time: 2 minutes

Cooking Time: 15 minutes

Serving: 2

Ingredients:

- 2 tbsp. extra-virgin olive oil, divided
- 2 lb. chuck roast, cut into 2" cubes
- Kosher salt
- Freshly ground black pepper
- 1 medium yellow onion, chopped
- 5 cloves garlic, thinly sliced
- 1/2 tsp. fennel seeds
- 1/4 tsp. red pepper flakes
- 2 tbsp. tomato paste

- 1/4 c. red wine
- 1 (28 oz.) can whole peeled tomatoes
- 1/4 c. water
- 3 sprigs thyme
- 1 bay leaf
- 2 tsp. balsamic vinegar
- Parmesan, for serving
- Freshly chopped parsley, for serving

Direction:

1. Using stock pot over medium heat, heat 1 tablespoon oil. Sprinkle chuck roast with salt and pepper and sear for 10 minutes. Transfer into a large bowl.

2. Cook remaining oil at medium heat. Cook onion for 6 minutes. Stir-fry garlic, fennel seeds, and red pepper flakes for 1 minute more.

3. Pour in tomato paste and cook for 3 minutes more. Deglaze pot with wine

4. Mix in whole peeled tomatoes, water, thyme, bay leaf, balsamic vinegar, and seared pot roast and season well. Stir and set heat to low. Cover and simmer, stirring occasionally, for 2 1/2 hours. With a wooden spoon to break up tomatoes and meat, and remove bay leaf. Serve with parmesan and parsley before serving.

Nutrition: 180 Calories 14.1g Total fat 13.8g Carbohydrates

Blueberry Pancakes

Preparation Time: 5 minutes

Cooking Time: 15 minutes

Servings: 1

Ingredients:

- 2 cups all-purpose flour
- 2 tablespoons baking powder
- 1 teaspoon kosher salt
- 3 tablespoons light brown sugar
- 2 eggs
- 1 teaspoon vanilla
- 1 1/2 cups milk
- 5 tablespoons butter, melted
- 2 cups fresh blueberries
- butter for frying

Directions:

1. Incorporate flour, baking powder, salt and brown sugar together.
2. Scourge eggs, vanilla and milk together.
3. Pour in wet ingredients into the dry and mix until just combined. Lastly stir in the melted butter. Put the batter aside while preheating the griddle to medium-low heat. Cook small pat of butter on the griddle then spoon out

1/4 cup of batter onto the hot griddle then top evenly with blueberries.

4. Cook and flip until browned.

5. Serve warm.

Nutrition: 45 Calories 0.1g Total fat 11.9g Carbohydrates

Brown Sugar Bacon

Preparation Time: 5 minutes

Cooking Time: 20 minutes

Servings: 11

Ingredients:

- 1/4 cup firmly packed brown sugar
- 8 slices thick-cut bacon
- 2 teaspoons chili powder

Direction:

1. Set oven to 400F. Prep rimmed baking sheet with aluminum foil. Situate cooling rack inside the prepared pan and set aside.
2. Mix brown sugar and chili powder. Crumble bacon slices in the brown sugar mixture and situate the bacon on the rack. Bake for 20 minutes. Serve.

Nutrition: 157 Calories 3g Carbohydrates 11g Protein

Starbucks Pumpkin Bread

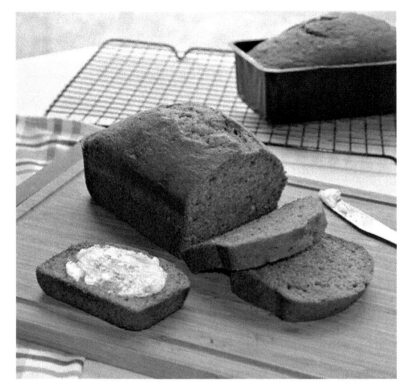

Preparation Time: 15 minutes

Cooking Time: 1 hour and 10 minutes

Servings: 11

Ingredients:

- 1 ½ cups all-purpose flour
- 1 teaspoon baking soda
- 1 teaspoon ground nutmeg
- 1 teaspoon ground cinnamon
- 1 teaspoon ground cloves

- ½ teaspoon baking powder
- ½ teaspoon salt
- 4 large eggs
- 1 cup white sugar
- ¼ cup light brown sugar
- ½ teaspoon vanilla extract
- ¾ cup canned pumpkin
- ¾ cup vegetable oil

Directions:

1. Prep oven to 350 degrees F (175 degrees C). Brush 8-1/2x4-1/2-inch loaf pan.
2. Incorporate flour, baking soda, nutmeg, cinnamon, cloves, baking powder, and salt
3. Scourge eggs, white sugar, brown sugar, and vanilla extract using electric mixer on high speed for 30 seconds. Stir in pumpkin and oil. Mix flour mixture
4. Pour batter into the prepared loaf pan. Bake for 70 minutes. Set aside in the pan for 30 minutes. Reverse onto a wire rack and cut it into 1-inch-thick slices.

Nutrition: 429.6 Calories 23.6g Total fat 50.1g Carbohydrates

APPETIZER RECIPES

Copycat California Pizza Kitchen's California Club Pizza

Preparation Time: 5 minutes

Cooking Time: 12 minutes

Serving: 4

Ingredients

- 1 ball pizza dough
- 2 tablespoons olive oil
- 1 chicken breast
- 4 slices of bacon
- 1 cup mozzarella cheese, grated
- 1½ cups arugula
- 2 tablespoons mayonnaise
- 1 tomato, sliced
- 1 avocado

Direction

1. Preheat pizza stone in oven to 425°F.
2. Using a rolling pin, flatten pizza dough until it is about 12 to 14 inches in diameter. Brush olive oil in a thin and

even layer on top. Add chicken, bacon, and mozzarella in layers evenly across pizza dough.

3. Place onto pizza stone and bake for about 10 to 12 minutes or until cheese melts and crust is slightly brown. Remove from oven and set aside.

4. In a bowl, add arugula and mayonnaise. Mix well. Top cooked pizza with tomato, arugula mixture, and avocado.

5. Serve warm.

Nutrition: 456 Calories 32g Fats 26g Protein

Taco Bell's Mexican Pizza

Preparation Time: 27 minutes

Cooking Time: 13 minutes

Serving: 3

Ingredients

- ½ lb. ground beef
- ½ tsp. salt
- ¼ tsp. onion
- ¼ tsp. paprika
- 1½ tsp. chili powder
- 2 tbsp. water
- 1 cup vegetable oil
- 8 6-inch flour tortillas
- 1 16-oz can refry beans
- 2/3 cup picante sauce
- 1/3 cup tomato
- 1 cup cheddar cheese
- 1 cup Colby jack cheese
- ¼ cup green onion
- ¼ cup black olives

Direction

1. Prep oven to 400°F.

2. Using a skillet, cook beef on medium heat. When brown, strain. Sprinkle salt, onions, paprika, chili powder, and water. Continue stirring, cook for extra 10 minutes.

3. In a different skillet, pour oil and heat at medium-high. Warm up tortilla for 30 seconds on both sides. Prick any bubbles forming on the tortillas. Situate onto a plate lined with paper towels.

4. Reheat the refried beans on high until warm.

5. To build each pizza, brush 1/3 cup beans on tortilla then 1/3 cup cooked beef. Place a second tortilla. Spread 2 tablespoons picante sauce, and equal amounts of tomatoes, cheeses, green onions, and olives.

6. Situate prepared pizzas on baking sheet. Bake for 11 minutes.

Nutrition: 217 Calories 87g Fats 31g Protein

Copycat Cici's Spinach-Alfredo Pizza

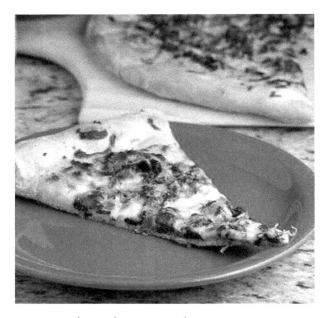

Preparation Time: 10 minutes

Cooking Time: 20 minutes

Serving: 6

Ingredients

- 2 tablespoons butter
- ½ teaspoon salt
- ¼ teaspoon black pepper
- ¾ cup heavy cream
- 3 ounces Romano cheese, shredded
- 1 pizza crust
- ½ package frozen spinach, thawed and drained

- 8 ounces mozzarella cheese, grated

Direction

1. Preheat oven to 450°F.

2. Prepare Alfredo sauce by adding butter to a deep pan over medium heat. Once melted, add salt, pepper, and heavy cream. Bring to boil while stirring frequently. Remove from heat. Once sauce has cooled a bit, stir in Romano cheese until melted.

3. Place pizza crust onto a baking tray. Thinly coat Alfredo sauce on crust then spread spinach over sauce. Sprinkle mozzarella evenly on top.

4. Bake for 13 minutes.

5. Serve.

Nutrition: 334 Calories 28g Fats 14g Protein

Domino's Philly Cheese Steak Pizza

Preparation Time: 60 minutes

Cooking Time: 3 hours

Serves: 8

Ingredients:

- Use recipe for Dominos-style hand tossed crust scale down for one pizza
- 1/2 cup provolone cheese
- 3/4 cup American cheese
- 6 ounces mushrooms
- 1 medium white onion
- 1 medium green bell pepper
- 1/3-pound deli roast beef
- 3 tablespoons olive oil
- Salt and pepper to taste

Direction

1. Create hand-tossed dough recipe up until the kneading process.
2. Stir in provolone cheese, and continue recipe until dough is ready to bake.
3. Prep the oven to 500 degrees.
4. Using a skillet, heat oil over medium-high heat.

5. Fry peppers, onions and mushrooms to the skillet for 15 minutes.

6. Add the roast beef pieces, and sauté until heated through. Drain.

7. Season well

8. Arrange vegetable and steak mixture over the top of the pizza dough.

9. Drizzle with provolone and American cheeses.

10. Bake for 11 minutes. Set aside. Slice into 8 pieces and serve.

Nutrition: 334 Calories 28g Fats 14g Protein

Papa John's Chicken Bacon Ranch Pizza

Preparation Time: 30 minutes

Cooking Time: 20 minutes

Serving: 4

Ingredients:

- 1 8oz can pizza dough OR use Papa John's Original Crust Recipe
- 2 cups cooked chicken breast halves (chopped)
- 8 slices cooked bacon (cut up)
- 1/4 cup red onion (chopped)
- 1 1/2 cups pre-shredded mozzarella cheese

Sauce:

- 1/3-1/2 cup ranch dressing
- 1/4 cup butter
- 1 1/2 ounces cream cheese
- 1/2-pint heavy whipping cream
- 1/2 teaspoon garlic powder
- 1/4 cup grated parmesan cheese
- Salt and black pepper

Directions:

1. Set oven to 425F. Spread out pizza dough onto your pizza pan or cookie sheet.

2. Prep sauce. Using saucepan over low heat, melt butter. Mix in the cream cheese. Stir in the cream and garlic powder.

3. Increase the heat and boil. Reduce the heat and simmer.

4. If it's too thin, stir in some flour 1 teaspoon at a time. Cook and stir for desired consistency.

5. Drizzle in the parmesan cheese and season well.

6. Lay out your ranch dressing on your dough first, next spread your alfredo sauce on the dough.

7. Drizzle half of your mozzarella cheese on the pizza.

8. Mix in shredded chicken, bacon and chopped onion.

9. Drizzle remaining cheese and bake at 425 on the bottom rack of oven for 20 minutes. Serve

Nutrition: 334 Calories 28g Fats 14g Protein

Papa John's Chocolate Chip Pizza Cookie

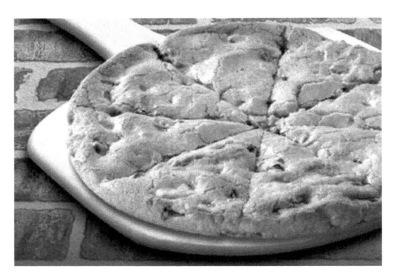

Preparation Time: 12 minutes

Cooking Time: 39 minutes

Serving: 4

Ingredients:

- 2 cups all-purpose flour
- 1 tsp. salt
- 1 tsp. baking powder
- 1 cups butter, softened
- 1 cup dark brown sugar
- 1 cup granulated sugar
- 2 eggs

- 1 cups chocolate chip, semisweet

Direction

1. Incorporate flour, baking powder and salt and put aside.

2. Beat butter with the granulated sugar.

3. Scourge eggs and brown sugar into the butter mixture.

4. Transfer wet ingredients into the dry ingredients and combine until they form a sticky cookie dough.

5. Stir in the chocolate chips last.

6. Prep a 12-inch pie pan by lining it with parchment paper.

7. Arrange cookie dough evenly in the pie pan so that it reaches all sides.

8. Bake the cookie at 350F for 17 minutes.

Nutrition: 374 Calories 21g Fats 11g Protein

Pizza Hut's Salted Pretzel Pizza Crust

Preparation time: 30 minutes

Cooking time: 20 minutes

Serving: 4

Ingredients:

- 1-1/3 cups warm water
- 1 tablespoon active dry yeast
- 2 tablespoons honey
- 3-1/2 cups all-purpose flour
- 1 teaspoon salt (regular fine table salt)
- 1/3 cup baking soda
- 1 tablespoon melted butter
- Coarse sea salt
- 1 cup pizza sauce
- 1 cup shredded cheese
- Pepperoni slices or other desired toppings

Direction

1. Mix warm water, yeast, and honey and stir to mix.
2. Set aside for 5 minutes
3. Stir flour and 1 teaspoon salt to yeast mixture. Mix until a dough form.
4. Knead until dough is tacky but not too sticky.

5. Take dough from bowl and allow to rest on a well-floured surface for 10 minutes.

6. Fill a stock pot with about 2-3 inches of water.

7. Boil water and sprinkle baking soda. Decrease water to a simmer.

8. Portion dough into three equal portions and roll them out into three 8-inch discs.

9. Mildly drop one dough disc into the simmering water. Allow to boil for 30-40 seconds.

10. Use slotted spoons, carefully lift dough from the pot and transfer to a paper-towel lined cooling rack. Do with remaining two dough discs.

11. Situate dough discs to a greased baking sheet

12. Brush with melted butter. Season with coarse sea salt. Bake for 10 minutes at 420F. Garnish with pizza sauce, cheese, and pepperoni.

13. Bake for 10-15 minutes more. Serve immediately.

Nutrition: 384 Calories 24g Fats 10g Protein

Domino's Crunchy Thin Crust

Preparation Time: 35 minutes

Cooking Time: 26 minutes

Serving: 8

Ingredients:

- 1 3/4 cup high-gluten wheat flour
- 1/2 cup warm water
- 1 tablespoon soybean oil (or other vegetable oil)
- 3/4 teaspoon active yeast
- 1 1/2 teaspoon sugar
- 1/4 teaspoon salt
- 3/4 cup pizza sauce
- 1 cup whole milk mozzarella cheese, shredded

Direction

1. Preheat the oven to 500 degrees.
2. Mix together the water, yeast, sugar, salt and oil until the powder ingredients are completely dissolved.
3. Stir in flour and mix on low speed with a dough mixer until a ball form.
4. Pull out dough from the bowl, and place on a floured surface.
5. Knead until the dough is elastic and still a bit moist.
6. Situate dough between two pieces of parchment paper.

7. Use a rolling pin to flatten the dough into a circle 1/4-inch thick.

8. Bake the crust for four minutes, then remove from the oven.

9. Spread pizza sauce evenly over the pizza.

10. Top with cheese and any other topping choices.

11. Bake for five minutes. Then rotate, and bake or an additional five or six minutes.

12. Pull out pizza from the oven and set aside for five minutes.

13. Slice into eight pieces and serve.

Nutrition: 364 Calories 25g Fats 8g Protein

Papa John's Original Crust

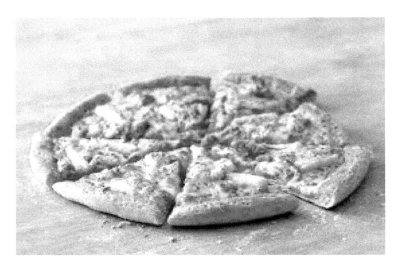

Preparation Time: 10 minutes

Cooking Time: 35 minutes

Serving: 4

Ingredients:

- 3 cups flour
- 2 tbsp. sugar
- 2 ¼ tsp. fast rising yeast
- 1/2 tsp. salt
- 1 cup very warm water
- 2 tbsp. oil

Direction

1. Mix 1 cup flour, sugar, undissolved yeast, and salt; blend well.

2. Gradually pour in water and oil to mixture.

3. Mix at low speed until moistened, then beat for 2 minutes at medium speed.

4. Mix in 2 cups flour until dough pulls away from sides of bowl.

5. On floured surface, knead in 1/2 cup flour until dough is smooth and elastic.

6. Seal loosely with plastic and set aside in a warm place for about 15 minutes.

7. Pound dough onto (2) 12-inch pizza pans.

8. Poke randomly with a fork. Keep aside in a warm place for 10-15 minutes.

9. Grease crusts lightly with oil then prebake them in a 450-degree oven for 5 minutes.

10. Top as desired, then bake again in 450F oven for 4-5 minutes.

Nutrition: 374 Calories 27g Fats 9g Protein

SOUP RECIPES

Egg and Pork Curry Soup with Udon Noodles

Preparation Time: 10 minutes

Cooking Time: 50 minutes

Servings: 4

Ingredients:

- One tablespoon of sunflower oil
- Half a cup of unsalted butter
- Two green shallots (long, shredded green parts, chopped white parts)
- Two-thirds cup of plain flour
- Eight cups of beef stock
- 1.5 tablespoons of curry powder
- One teaspoon of dark soy sauce
- One tablespoon each of
- Sake
- Mirin
- Four eggs (must be kept at room temperature)
- Five ounces of udon noodles

- For serving – bonito flakes and nori sheets
- For the pork,
- Two tablespoons of sake
- Two teaspoons of raw sugar
- One tablespoon each of
- Dark soy sauce
- Mirin
- 1.5 inches of ginger (grated finely)
- Two tablespoons of sunflower oil
- 17.5 ounces of minced pork

Directions:

1. Heat the stock and keep it aside. Take another saucepan and, in it, heat the oil—Cook the shallots for about three minutes. Then, add butter and stir. Stir in flour and cook for another three minutes.

2. Add curry powder and keep stirring for a minute. Then, add the hot stock into the mixture. If you can't add it at once, then add it in batches. Simmer. Add sake, soy sauce, and mirin, and mix them well in the soup.

3. It is time to prepare the pork. Heat the oil. Add ginger and pork and break the pork with the help of a spoon.

Keep cooking for five minutes. Incorporate the rest of the ingredients and cook for another three minutes.

4. Add water to another saucepan and boil the water. Add the eggs and cook them to your liking. Drain the water and keep the eggs in another bowl. Peel once it cools down.

5. Boil the soup again. Take the serving bowls and divide the soup and noodles evenly. Top the soup with halved eggs, pork mixture, nori, shredded shallot, and bonito. Serve.

Nutrition: 508 Calories 23.9g Protein 14.3g Fat

Curry Udon Noodles

Preparation Time: 15 minutes

Cooking Time: 40 minutes

Servings: 2

Ingredients:

- One spring onion
- 760ml water
- Four tablespoons of tsuyu soup stock
- Two packets of udon noodles (pre-cooked)
- Half each of Carrot, Potato and Onion
- Three blocks of Japanese curry roux

Directions:

1. Add 360ml of water to a pan. Chop the carrot, potato, and onion into small pieces and add them to the pan. Bring it to a boil. Simmer until the vegetables soften, for about 20 minutes.

2. Add three blocks of curry roux and simmer for ten minutes. Stir continuously until the curry sauce is smooth and thick.

3. Take a separate pan, add 400ml of water, and add four tbsp of tsuyu soup stock for making the noodle soup. Boil it. Boil the udon noodles and drain them after a few minutes in the colander.

4. Take a bowl and place the udon noodles, pour the noodle soup, pour the curry sauce on top. Topped with some sliced spring onions.

Nutrition: 340 Calories 7g Protein 14g Fat

Kitsune Udon

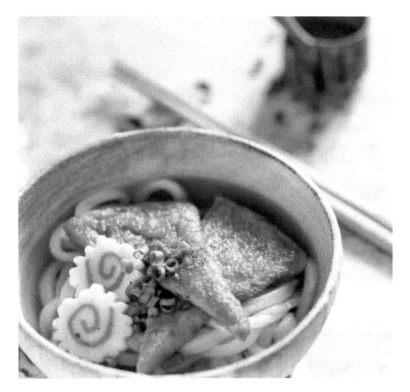

Preparation Time: 15 minutes

Cooking Time: 50 minutes

Servings: 2

Ingredients:

- Four pouches of Inari Age
- Two servings of udon noodles
- One scallion or green onion, sliced thinly
- One tablespoon each of
- Usukuchi soy sauce

- Mirin
- Two and a quarter cups of dashi
- One teaspoon of sugar
- Shichimi Togarashi (optional)
- Narutomaki (optional), cut into 1/8-inch pieces

For the homemade dashi,

- One and a half cups of katsuobushi
- One kombu
- Two and a half cups of water

Directions:

1. You can use store-bought dashi powder or make it on your own. To make the homemade dashi, add the kombu in two and a half cups of water then soak for 30 minutes. You can also soak it for three hours or up to half a day as it helps bring out the flavor of the kombu.

2. Add the kombu and water into a saucepan and boil it over medium-low heat. Discard the kombu just before the water starts boiling. The dashi will turn bitter and slimy if you keep the kombu in the water for too long while it is boiling.

3. Add in one and a half cups of katsuobushi and boil again. Lower the heat when the dashi is boiling and let it simmer for fifteen minutes and then turn off the heat. Allow the katsuobushi to sink to the bottom of the pan

and then keep it for ten to fifteen minutes. Use a fine-mesh sieve to strain the dashi into a saucepan. Your homemade dashi is now ready.

4. Add the soy sauce, sugar, mirin, dashi, and salt into a saucepan and boil the mixture. Then, cover or turn off the heat and let it simmer.

5. Add the udon noodles into a large pot of water and boil it. Once it gets cooked, transfer it into a strainer and drain all the water.

6. Add the soup and the udon noodles equally into serving bowls and add the shichimi togarashi, green onions, narutomaki, and Inari Age as a garnish.

Nutrition: 413 Calories 10g Protein 15.5g Fat

Momofuku Soy Sauce Eggs, Chili Chicken, and Soba Noodles

Preparation Time: 15 minutes

Cooking Time: 30 minutes

Servings: 4

Ingredients:

- 3.5 ounces of enoki mushrooms, trimmed
- One toasted nori sheet, torn
- 1.5 ounces of soba noodles, cooked and refreshed
- Four eggs, hard-boiled and peeled
- Three cups of chicken stock
- One-third of a cup of white miso paste
- One teaspoon each of
- Ginger, finely grated
- Chili garlic paste
- Four spring onions, thinly sliced and some extra shredded onions for serving
- 7 ounces of chicken, minced
- Two teaspoons of olive oil (extra virgin)
- One cup Soy sauce
- One cup Rice wine vinegar
- Shichimi togarashi, to serve

Directions:

1. Keep the eggs, soy sauce, and vinegar in a non-reactive bowl and chill overnight or for three to four hours.

2. Situate frying pan over high heat and add one teaspoon of oil in it. Then add the minced chicken and cook for five minutes and break the pieces using a wooden spoon. Add in the chili garlic paste when the chicken turns brown and cook for another three to four minutes so that they get brownish. Keep warm.

3. Place a saucepan over medium-low heat and heat the remaining teaspoon of oil in it. Add in the ginger and onions and cook for three to four minutes and occasionally stir so that they get tender. Pour in the stock and miso and stir so that the miso dissolves.

4. Divide the nori, soup, and noodles among serving bowls. Add the extra onion, mushroom, halved eggs and mince mixture as a topping. Sprinkle some shichimi togarashi and serve.

Nutrition: 443.3 Calories 40g Protein 16g Fat

Soba, Prawn, and Lemongrass Soup

Preparation Time: 15 minutes

Cooking Time: 1 hour and 20 minutes

Servings: 4

Ingredients:

- Six ounces of dried soba noodles
- 5 ounces of king prawns (medium-sized), peeled and deveined with the tails intact
- Eight cups of chicken stock
- 6-inch piece of lemongrass (only the white part), cut in half lengthwise
- 1.5-inch of ginger, thinly sliced
- Two eschalots, thinly sliced
- Two teaspoons Sesame oil
- Two teaspoon Soy sauce
- Two green shallots, thinly sliced
- One red chili, thinly sliced
- One teaspoon Sesame seeds
- One teaspoon Rice vinegar
- Mirin

Directions:

1. Situate a big saucepan over medium-high heat and heat some sesame oil in it. Add in the ginger and eschalots

and cook for three to four minutes so that the eschalots get tender. Add in the chicken stock and lemongrass and boil the mixture. Lower the heat to low and let it simmer for thirty-five to forty minutes.

2. Mix in the prawns and cook for extra two to three minutes. Then, add the vinegar, mirin, soy, and noodles and stir. Garnish with green shallots, chili, and sesame seeds.

Nutrition: 180.6 Calories 20g Protein 0.3g Fat

Ancient Grains Soup

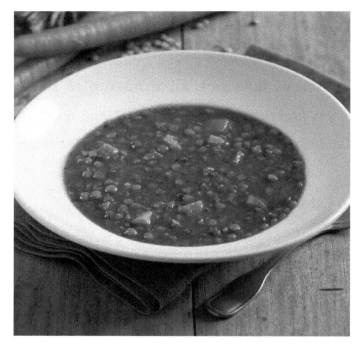

Preparation Time: 10 minutes

Cooking Time: 45 minutes

Servings: 6

Ingredients

- 1 ¾ ounces celery, diced
- 2 ½ ounces onion, diced
- 1 teaspoon fresh parsley, chopped
- 2 ½ ounces carrot, peeled & diced
- 1 ½ ounces freekeh, cooked
- 2 teaspoon garlic, crushed (approximately 2 cloves)

- 1 can tomatoes, chopped (1 pound)
- 2 ounces amaranth, cooked
- 1 ½ ounces quinoa, cooked
- ¾ tablespoon olive oil
- 14 ounces water
- ¼ teaspoon each of pepper & salt

Directions

1. Over moderate heat in a medium casserole; heat the olive oil for a couple of minutes. Once hot; add & cook the onion together with celery, garlic, and carrot until for 3 to 5 minutes, until onion is translucent.

2. Add tomatoes (along with its accumulated juices) followed by freekeh, amaranth, quinoa & water. Adjust the heat then boil mixture. Once done; decrease the heat & let simmer for 12 to 15 more minutes then, remove the casserole from heat.

3. Carefully situate the contents to a blender & add in the parsley. Purée until combined well. Season with pepper and salt. Serve hot & enjoy.

Nutrition 171 calories 28g carbs 26g protein

Piranha Pale Ale Chili

Preparation Time: 40 minutes

Cooking Time: 40 minutes

Servings: 8

Ingredients

- 1 lb. each of ground beef & ground pork
- 2 tablespoons chili powder
- 1 bottle Piranha Pale Ale (12-ounce)
- 2 cups onion, diced
- 1 teaspoon ground black pepper
- ½ teaspoon cayenne
- 1 teaspoon garlic powder
- 2 cups water
- 1 can crushed tomatoes (15-ounce)
- ½ cup all-purpose flour
- 1 teaspoon dried thyme
- 2 cans pinto beans (15-ounce, along with the liquid)
- 1 tablespoon salt

For Garnish:

- 1 cups cheddar cheese, shredded
- ½ cup sour cream
- 1 cup Monterey Jack cheese, shredded

- ½ cup green onion, chopped

Directions

1. Brown the ground meats over medium heat in a large saucepan. Drain any excess fat off. Add onion followed by cayenne, garlic powder, chili powder, spices, black pepper, thyme, and salt; continue to sauté for 3 to 5 more minutes.

2. Combine flour with water & add the mixture to the pan.

3. Add the leftover ingredients to the hot pan; bring the chili to a simmer & let simmer for 1 ½ hours, uncovered, stirring occasionally.

4. Serve approximately 1 ¼ cups of the prepared chili in a carved-out round of sourdough bread or in a bowl. Combine the shredded cheeses together & top the chili with approximately ¼ cup of the cheese blend followed by a tablespoon of the sour cream & garnish with a tablespoon of chopped green onions. Serve and enjoy.

Nutrition: 175 calories 30g carbs 24g protein

Chicken Tortilla Soup

Preparation Time: 9 minutes

Cooking Time: 34 minutes

Servings: 3

Ingredients

- ½ cup sweet corn
- 1 cup onion
- 3 tbsp. fresh cilantro
- 1 cup chicken broth
- 1 chicken breast
- Avocado to taste
- 1 (8 oz.) can chilies & tomatoes
- 1 lime juice
- 1 cup water

Directions

1. At moderate heat in a deep pot; mix chicken broth together with water, onion, chili and tomatoes, corn and cilantro; boil and stirring occasionally. Stir in the chicken pieces; stir and reduce heat to simmer. Cook for extra minutes, until cooked through. Mix in Tortilla chips followed by avocado & cheese to taste in serving bowls. Pour the soup & drizzle lime juice. Serve

Nutrition: 175 calories 44g carbs 31g protein

Tuscan Tomato Bisque

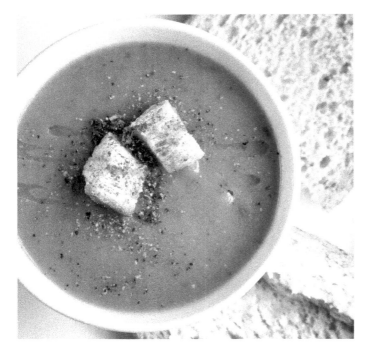

Preparation

Time: 10 minutes

Cooking Time: 20 minutes

Servings: 4

Ingredients

- 4 garlic cloves, crushed
- 1 can chicken broth (14 ½ ounce), undiluted
- 2 cans no-salt-added diced tomatoes (14 ½ ounce each), undrained
- 1 teaspoon olive oil
- 4 -5 teaspoons parmesan cheese, grated

- 1 tablespoon balsamic vinegar
- 2 ½ cups 1" French bread cubes (2 ½ slices)
- 1 ½ teaspoons parsley flakes, dried
- Olive oil flavored cooking spray
- 1 teaspoon oregano, dried
- ½ teaspoon pepper

Directions

1. Situate bread cubes on a baking sheet in 1 layer & coat the bread lightly with the cooking spray.
2. Bake until dry & toasted, for 8 to 10 minutes, at 400 F.
3. Now, over medium-low heat in large saucepan; heat the olive oil.
4. Once hot; add and sauté the garlic for 2 minutes.
5. Add the leftover ingredients (except grated parmesan cheese) & bring the mixture to a boil.
6. Decrease the heat & let simmer for 10 minutes, stirring every now and then.
7. Evenly divide the croutons among 4 to 5 bowls; ladle the soup over & sprinkle with the grated parmesan cheese. Serve immediately & enjoy.

Nutrition: 166 calories 31g carbs 22g protein

Broccoli Cheddar Soup

Preparation Time: 20 minutes

Cooking Time: 40 minutes

Servings: 4

Ingredients

- 6 tablespoons unsalted butter
- 1 small onion, chopped
- 2 cups half-and-half
- ¼ cup all-purpose flour
- 3 cups chicken broth, low-sodium
- ¼ teaspoon nutmeg, freshly grated
- 4 (7" each) sourdough bread boules (round loaves)
- 2 bay leaves
- 4 cups broccoli florets (1 large head)
- 2 ½ cups (approximately 8 ounces) sharp white & yellow cheddar cheese, grated, plus more for garnish
- 1 large carrot, diced
- Freshly ground pepper & kosher salt to taste

Directions

1. Over moderate heat in a large pot or Dutch oven; heat the butter until melted. Add and cook the onion for 3 to 5 minutes, until tender. Whisk in the flour & continue to cook for 3 to 4 more minutes, until turn golden. Slowly

whisk in the half-and-half until completely smooth. Add the chicken broth followed by nutmeg and bay leaves, then season with pepper and salt; bring the mixture to a simmer. Once done; decrease the heat to medium-low & cook for 15 to 20 more minutes, until thickened, uncovered.

2. In the meantime, prepare the bread bowls: Cut a circle into the top of each loaf using a sharp knife, leaving approximately 1" border all around. Remove the bread top and then hollow out the middle using your fingers or with a fork, leaving a thick bread shell.

3. Add the carrot & broccoli to the broth mixture & let simmer for 15 to 20 minutes, until tender. Discard the bay leaves. Work in batches & carefully puree the soup in a blender until smooth. Add to the pot again.

4. Add the cheese to the soup & continue to whisk over medium heat until melted. If the soup appears to be too thick; feel free to add up to ¾ cup of water. Ladle into the bread bowls & garnish with cheese. Serve immediately & enjoy.

Nutrition: 178 calories 33g carbs 25g protein

MAIN RECIPES

Chicken and Asparagus

Preparation Time: 5 minutes

Cooking Time: 20 minutes

Servings: 4

Ingredients:

- 4 chicken breasts, skinless; boneless and halved
- 1 bunch asparagus; trimmed and halved
- 1 tbsp. olive oil
- 1 tbsp. sweet paprika
- Salt and black pepper to taste.

Directions:

1. Begin by cooking the aromatics: I incorporate the regular onions, celery and carrots. Sauté those until they're fragrant and fork delicate but not as well soft. Add within the flavoring you're utilizing. I keep it straightforward with salt, pepper, garlic and oregano. Then include the tomatoes. I utilize a combination of diced canned tomatoes and tomato paste. Particle. But you'll too use fresh tomatoes and tomato sauce or any other variety to

urge a tomato broth. Add vegetable broth, chicken broth or hamburger broth and bring to a boil. Finally include the cabbage and cook until the cabbage shrivels, around 20 minutes.

Nutrition: 230 Calories 11g Fat 12g Protein

Basil Chicken Bites

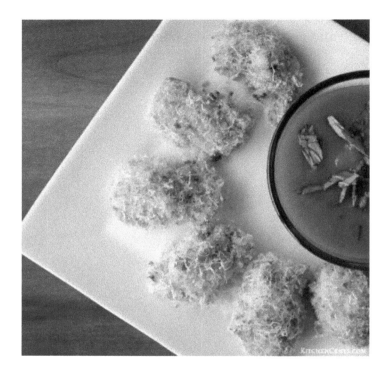

Preparation Time: 10 minutes

Cooking Time: 25 minutes

Servings: 4

Ingredients:

- 1 ½ lb. chicken breasts, skinless; boneless and cubed
- ½ cup chicken stock
- ½ tsp. basil; dried
- 2 tsp. smoked paprika
- Salt and black pepper to taste.

Directions:

1. Combine ingredients in a huge bowl. Let marinate for 10 minutes. Heat oil in a deep-fryer or expansive pan to 400 degrees F (200 degrees C). Whisk egg in a little bowl until smooth. Pour tempura player blend into a moment little bowl. Plunge chicken pieces one at a time into the egg, at that point dig in tempura player blend, shaking off any abundance. Situate chicken pieces carefully into the hot oil in batches. Sear until chicken is brilliant brown, 5 to 8 minutes.

2. Serve chicken sprinkled with basil leaves, green onions, white pepper, and salt.

Nutrition: 223 Calories 12g Fat 13g Protein

BBQ Beef Brisket Sandwiches

Preparation Time: 15 minutes

Cooking Time: 9 hours and 5 minutes

Serving: 4

Ingredients

- 1 ½ lb. beef brisket
- 1 teaspoon celery salt
- 1 teaspoon of black pepper
- ½ cup Russian sauce
- ¾ teaspoon salt, or to taste
- ½ teaspoon garlic powder
- ½ teaspoon onion salt
- 1 teaspoon Worcestershire sauce
- ½ cup of barbecue sauce, walnut flavored

Directions

1. Combine celery salt, salt, black pepper, garlic, and onion salt in a clean small bowl; add Worcestershire sauce;
2. Spread the mixture over the ox breast; transfer to a slow cooker;
3. Cook over low heat until meat is tender, about 8 hours;
4. Transfer the cooked tender meat to a cutting board; shred in small pieces using two forks;

5. Measure ½ cup of the slow cooker in a saucepan. Mix Russian sauce and barbecue sauce; let it boil;

6. Combine the meat mixture and grated sauce in a slow cooker;

7. Cook over low heat until the flavors combine, about 1 hour.

Nutrition: 36g Carbohydrates 4g Fat 106 Calories

Mongolian Meat

Preparation Time: 10 minutes

Cooking Time: 15 minutes

Serving: 4

Ingredients

- 1 lb. flank steak
- ¼ cup cornstarch
- ¼ cup canola oil
- 2 teaspoons fresh ginger, chopped
- 1 tablespoon garlic, chopped
- 1/3 Cup soy sauce, low sodium
- 1/3 Cup of water
- ½ cup dark brown sugar
- 4 green onion stalks, only green parts, cut into 2" pieces

Directions

1. Slice flank steak against the grain along the ¼" reflection pieces and add it to a zippered pouch with cornstarch;
2. Press the steak into the bag, making sure that each piece is completely covered with cornstarch and let it rest;
3. Add canola oil to a considerable large skillet and heat over medium-high heat;
4. Add the steak, shaking off the excess cornstarch, to the pan in a single layer, and cook per side for 1 minute;

5. If you have to cook the steak in batches because your pan is not big enough, make it instead of cluttering it, you want to have a good grip on the steak and fill the pot with steam instead of burning;

6. When the steak is cooked, remove it from the pan;

7. Stir in chopped ginger and garlic to the pan and sauté for 10-15 seconds;

8. Add the water, soy sauce, and dark brown sugar to the pan and cook it to a boil;

9. Add the steak and let the sauce thicken for 20 to 30 seconds;

10. The corn starch we use in the steak should thicken the sauce. If you realize that it is not thickening enough, add 1 tablespoon of corn starch to 1 tbsp. of cold water and stir to break up the corn starch and include it to the skillet;

11. Add the green onion, stir to combine, and cook for nearly 20 to 30 seconds;

12. Serve fresh immediately.

Nutrition: 143 calories 26g protein 4g fat

Parmesan Chicken

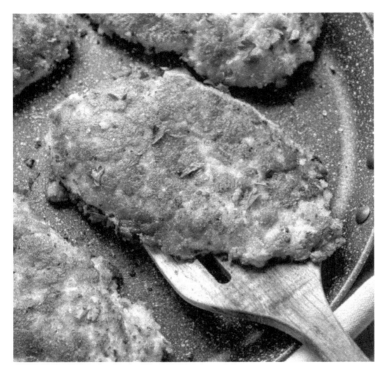

Preparation Time: 25 minutes

Cooking Time: 35 minutes

Serving: 4

Ingredients

- 4 boneless, skinless chicken breast halves
- Salt and black pepper to taste
- 2 eggs
- 1 cup panko breadcrumbs
- ½ cup of parmesan, grated

- 2 tablespoons of wheat flour
- 1 cup of cooking oil, for cooking
- ½ cup of tomato sauce
- ¼ cup fresh mozzarella, diced
- ¼ cup fresh basil, chopped
- ½ cup provolone cheese, grated
- ¼ cup of parmesan, grated
- 1 tablespoon of olive oil

Directions

1. Preheat an oven to 450° F;
2. The chicken breasts should be placed between two sheets of thick plastic (the resalable freezer bags work well) on a stable, level surface. Firmly grind the chicken with the smooth side of a meat mallet to a thickness of ½";
3. Season the chicken carefully with salt and pepper;
4. Beat the eggs in a considerable shallow bowl and set aside;
5. Mix breadcrumbs and ½ cup parmesan in another bowl, set aside;
6. Put the flour in a sieve; sprinkle over chicken breasts, evenly covering both sides;
7. Dip the floured chicken breast in the eggs, beaten;
8. Transfer the breast to the breadcrumb mixture by pressing the crumbs on both sides;

9. Repeat the procedure for each breast - reserve breaded chicken breasts for about 15 minutes;

10. Heat 1 cup of oil in a large skillet over medium-high heat until it begins to shine;

11. Cook the chicken for 4 minutes both sides. The chicken will finish roasting;

12. Set the chicken in an ovenproof dish and decorate each breast with approximately 1/3 cup of tomato sauce;

13. Layer each chicken breast with equivalent measures of mozzarella cheese, fresh basil, and provolone cheese;

14. Sprinkle 1-2 tablespoons of Parmesan cheese on top and sprinkle with 1 tablespoon of olive oil;

15. Bake well in a preheated oven until the cheese is golden and bubbly, and the chicken breasts are no longer pink in color in the center, 15 to 20 minutes. An instant-read thermometer inserted in the center must read at least 165° F.

Nutrition: 205 calories 14g protein 10g fat

Chicken with Buttermilk

Preparation Time: 30 minutes

Cooking Time: 2 hours

Serving: 4

Ingredients

Marinade

- ½ cup buttermilk –
- ½ teaspoon of red pepper
- ¼ teaspoon of salt
- ½ clove of garlic, chopped

Chicken

- 2 lbs. of boneless, skinless chicken breast
- 1/3 Cup of wheat flour
- 1 tablespoon of cornstarch
- ½ teaspoon of dried thyme
- ½ teaspoon of paprika ground
- Frying Oil

Directions

1. Set the chicken pieces in a large reusable food storage bag. Add all the ingredients for the marinade and refrigerate for at least 2 hours or overnight to marinate;

2. In a pie dish, mix the flour and all other chicken ingredients except oil. Heat about ½" of oil in a 12" skillet over medium-high heat;

3. Remove the chicken pieces from the marinade, some at a time, allowing the excess to drain;

4. Wrap the chicken in the flour mixture until it is well coated;

5. Add the chicken to the hot oil in a pan, a few pieces simultaneously

6. Cook at medium-high heat for 10 minutes. Discard the marinade

7. Discover the pot. Flip the chicken over. Cook for 5 to 8 minutes more. Drain the chicken over several layers of paper towels;

8. Serve hot or refrigerate and serve cold.

Nutrition: 27g fat 29g protein 225 calories

Pulled Pork Sandwich

Preparation Time: 45 minutes

Cooking Time: 6 hours

Servings: 4

Ingredients

Pork

- 6 tablespoons of paprika
- 3 tablespoons sugar, granulated
- 1 tablespoon of onion powder
- Salt and black pepper, ground, to taste
- 1 (10-12 lbs.) boneless pork shoulder, washed and dried
- 12 sweet hamburger buns, cut in half
- Coleslaw, to serve

Barbecue sauce

- 2 cups of ketchup
- ¼ cup lightly packaged brown sugar
- ¼ cup sugar, granulated
- Black pepper, ground, to taste
- 1 ½ teaspoon onion powder, granulated
- 1 ½ teaspoon mustard powder
- 2 tablespoons lemon juice
- 2 tablespoons Worcestershire sauce

- ½ cup apple cider vinegar
- 2 tablespoons light corn syrup

Directions

1. If using a gas grill, preheat on one side;
2. Place the wood chips soaked in a smoking box. After smoking, reduce the heat to maintain a temperature of 275° F and grill the pork, covered, at the cooler side of the gas grill;
3. Combine the paprika, sugar and onion powder in a bowl;
4. Transfer 3 tablespoons of seasoning to a separate bowl, add 2 tablespoons of salt and 3 tablespoons of pepper and massage over the pork;
5. Carefully cover with plastic wrap and cool in a refrigerator for at least 2 hours or more (reserve the remaining barbecue seasoning);
6. Immerse 6 cups of wood chips in water, about 15 minutes, then drain. Do not immerse not too much; otherwise, the wood will go out of the fire;
7. Fill a smoker or kettle with charcoal and light. When the coals are becoming white, spread them out with tongs - spread ½ cup of wood chips over the grill coals (use 1 cup for grilling). The grill temperature should be around 275° F;

8. Set the fat pork face down on a grill in the smoker or on the grill;

9. Carefully cover and cook, turning the pork every hour or so until a thermometer inserted in the center records 165° F, about 6 hours in total;

10. While the pork is cooking, add more charcoal and wood chips to keep the temperature between 250° F and 275° F and maintain the smoke level;

11. Meanwhile, whisk the ketchup, 1 cup of water, the 2 sugars, 1 ½ teaspoons of pepper, onion and mustard powder, lemon juice, Worcestershire sauce, vinegar, syrup of corn and 1 tablespoon of barbecue seasoning reserved in a pan over high heat;

12. Heat to the point of boiling, stirring, then low the heat and cook, uncovered, occasionally stirring, at least 2 hours;

13. Transfer the pork to a roasting pan (you'll want to pick up all the delicious juices) and let it sit until its cold enough to handle;

14. Undo it in small pieces, stack it on a platter and pour the juice from the pan on top;

15. Mount the pork on the bottom of the cake, paint with a little barbecue sauce, top it with coleslaw and cover with the top cake. The best sandwich ever!

Nutrition: 32g Carbohydrates 9g Fat 243 Calories

Mud Pie

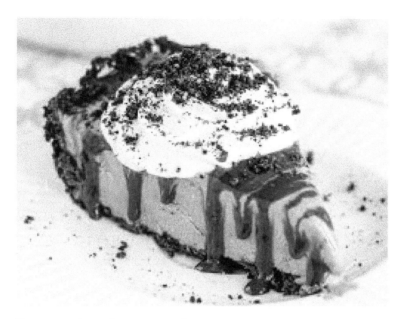

Preparation time: 30 minutes

Cooking Time: 15 minutes

Servings: 4

Ingredients

- ½ cup flour, all-purpose
- ½ cup chopped walnuts
- ¼ cup butter, softened
- ½ packet (3 oz.) of instant chocolate pudding mix
- ½ packet of cream cheese, softened
- ½ cup icing sugar
- ½ container (8 oz.) of frozen frosting

- Pecans and grated chocolate, to serve

Directions

1. Set the oven's temperature to exactly 350° F;
2. In a suitably large bowl, beat the flour, nuts, and butter until well combined;
3. Press the bottom of a 13X9" baking tray. Cook until golden brown, about 15 minutes;
4. Remove on a wire rack.
5. Create chocolate pudding following the package directions; let it sit and stand for 5 minutes.
6. Scourge cream cheese and sugar until smooth. Mix 1 cup of beaten frosting;
7. Spread the prepared cream cheese mixture on the cooled crust;
8. Spread the pudding on the cream cheese layer;
9. Decorate with the rest of the beaten frosting;
10. Decorate with additional chocolate chips and nuts if desired.

Nutrition: 20g Fat 6g Protein 146 Calories

DESSERT RECIPES

Cici's Apple Pizza

Preparation Time: 40 Minutes

Cooking Time: 30 Minutes

Servings: 8

Ingredients:

Crust

- 2 tablespoons sugar
- 1 tablespoon yeast
- 1½ cups warm water, about 105–110°F
- 4 tablespoons butter, softened
- 3 cups bread flour
- ½ teaspoon salt
  Apple Topping
- 1 (20-ounce) can apple pie filling
- 4 tablespoons butter, softened
- 2/3 cup brown sugar
- 2/3 cup bread flour
- 1 teaspoon cinnamon
  Glaze

- 1 tablespoon milk
- 1 teaspoon butter
- 2 cups powdered sugar

Directions:

1. Prepare the crust. Preheat oven to 350°F. In a mixer bowl, dissolve sugar and yeast in warm water. Add softened butter. Add the flour and salt. Using the dough hook, knead to make a smooth, sticky dough (about 5 minutes). Make it into a ball and let rest for 10 minutes. Roll out or press into a pizza pan. Through a fork to prick all over the surface. Bake for 15 minutes.

2. Prepare the topping. Chop the apple pieces. In a distinct bowl, combine the butter, brown sugar, bread flour and cinnamon to make a crumb topping.

3. Spread apple pie filling over baked crust and sprinkle evenly with crumb topping.

4. Bake until fragrant and lightly browned at the edges (about 10–15 minutes).

5. Prepare the glaze while the pie is baking. Place ingredients in a saucepan over low heat, stirring continuously until smooth. It should be a good constancy for drizzling. Add a few drops of water or milk if too thick.

6. Cool the pizza slightly (about 5 minutes) and then drizzle with glaze.

7. Let stand while glaze sets (about 5 minutes) and then serve.

Nutrition: Calories 149, Total Fat 3.6 g, Carbs 26.2 g, Protein 3 g, Sodium 0 mg

Taco Bell's Caramel Empanadas

Preparation Time: 20 Minutes

Cooking Time: 10 Minutes

Servings: 4

Ingredients:

- 1 tablespoon flour
- ¼ cup sugar
- 1 teaspoon cinnamon
- 4 medium apples, peeled, cored and diced
- ¼ cup water (optional).
- ¼ cup caramel sauce
- 2 tablespoons butter
- 2 premade pie crusts (dough)
- 1 egg white
- Oil, for frying (optional)
  Cinnamon Sugar Coating
- ¼ cup granulated sugar
- 1½ teaspoons cinnamon

Directions:

1. Preheat oven to 400°F.
2. Line a baking sheet with parchment paper.
3. Mix flour, sugar and cinnamon in a bowl. Set aside.

4. Place diced apples and water in a saucepan and bring to a boil. Decrease to a simmer and cook until apples are tender. Remove from heat. (If you prefer crisp apple in the filling, skip this step and eliminate water from recipe.)

5. Mix flour mixture into apples.

6. Add caramel sauce and butter. Set aside.

7. Take premade dough out of the refrigerator about 15 minutes before use. Roll out to about 10 inches in diameter. Use a bowl to cut out circles in the dough. Use a smaller bowl to make mini-empanadas.

8. Put filling into the center of each dough circle.

9. Brush egg white along the edges.

10. Fold the dough over like a turnover.

11. Press down on the edges by means of a fork, to seal.

12. Brush with egg white.

13. Combine ingredients for cinnamon sugar.

14. Sprinkle empanadas with cinnamon sugar and bake until golden brown (about 15 minutes).

15. The empanadas may also be deep fried (about 2–3 minutes on each side). Drain on paper towels and sprinkle cinnamon sugar after frying.

Nutrition: Calories 310, Total Fat 15 g, Carbs 39 g, Protein 3 g, Sodium 310 mg

Pizza Hut's Cherry Pizza

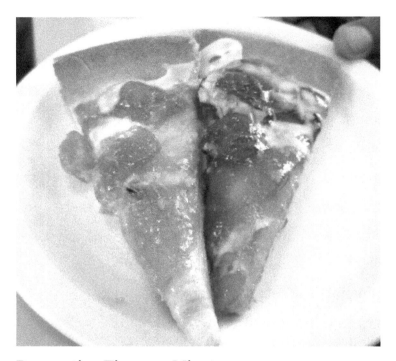

Preparation Time: 40 Minutes

Cooking Time: 30 Minutes

Servings: 8

Ingredients:

Crust

- 2 tablespoons sugar

- 1 tablespoon yeast

- 1½ cups warm water

- 4 tablespoons butter, softened

- 3 cups flour

- ½ teaspoon salt

  Cherry Topping and Streusel

- 1 (20-ounce) can cherry pie filling

- 4 tablespoons butter, softened

- 2/3 cup brown sugar

- 2/3 cup bread flour

- 1 teaspoon cinnamon

  Glaze

- 1 tablespoon milk

- 1 teaspoon of butter

- 2 cups powdered sugar

Directions:

1. Prepare the crust. Preheat oven to 350°F. In a mixer bowl, dissolve sugar and yeast in warm water. Add softened butter. Add the flour and salt. Using the dough hook, knead to make a smooth, sticky dough (about 5 minutes). Make into a ball and let rest for 10 minutes. Roll out or press into a pizza pan. Through a fork to prick all over the surface. Bake for 15 minutes.

2. Prepare the topping. Empty the can of cherry filling into a bowl and set aside. To make the streusel, combine the butter, brown sugar, bread flour and cinnamon in a separate bowl.

3. Spread cherry pie filling over baked crust and sprinkle evenly with the streusel.

4. Bake until fragrant and lightly browned at the edges (about 10–15 minutes).

5. Prepare the glaze while the pie is baking. Place ingredients in a saucepan over low heat, stirring continuously until smooth. It should be a good constancy for drizzling. Add a few drops of water or milk if too thick.

6. Cool the pizza slightly (about 5 minutes) and then drizzle with glaze.

7. Let stand to set glaze (about 5 minutes) and serve.

Nutrition: Calories 186, Total Fat 53 g, Carbs 32 g, Protein 1 g, Sodium 90 mg

Ruby Tuesday's Apple Pie

Preparation Time: 15 Minutes

Cooking Time: 60 Minutes

Servings: 8

Ingredients:

- 1 (9-inch) frozen apple pie
- ½ cup (1 stick) butter
- 1 cup brown sugar, packed, divided
- 3½ teaspoons cinnamon, divided
- ¼ teaspoon allspice
- ¼ teaspoon cloves
- 1½ teaspoons lemon juice
- ¾ cup flour
- ½ cup sugar
- 10 tablespoons frozen butter
- 1 cup chopped walnuts (optional)
- ½ gallon vanilla ice cream

Directions:

1. Allow pie to thaw as you prepare the other ingredients (about 30–45 minutes). Make a temporary hole in the pie by cutting an X in the center.
2. Preheat oven to 350°F.

3. Thaw butter in a saucepan over medium heat. Whisk in ½ cup brown sugar, 1½ teaspoons cinnamon, the allspice, cloves and lemon juice. As soon as sugar is fully dissolved, remove from heat.

4. Carefully open up the X in the pie by folding back the crust. Pour the butter mixture through the hole, slanting the pie from side to side to distribute the filling. Reseal the X and make a few small vent holes in the crust.

5. Bake for 30 minutes and remove from oven.

6. Turn oven temperature down to 325°F.

7. Wrap aluminum foil round the edge of the pie, to hold the topping.

8. Prepare the topping. Grate the frozen butter and toss with flour, remaining sugars, remaining cinnamon, and walnuts, if desired.

9. Sprinkle topping over pie.

10. Bake until filling is bubbling then crust is golden brown (about 30–40 minutes).

11. Remove from oven and let cool for 10–15 minutes.

12. Slice into wedges and serve with scoops of vanilla ice cream.

Nutrition: Calories 493, Total Fat 34 g, Carbs 46 g, Protein 4 g, Sodium 174 mg

Tommy Bahama's Key Lime Pie

Preparation Time: 40 Minutes

Cooking Time: 50 Minutes

Servings: 2

Ingredients:

Pie:

- 10-inch graham cracker crust
- 1 egg white
- 2½ cups sweetened condensed milk
- ¾ cup pasteurized egg yolk
- 1 cup lime juice
- 1 lime, zest
- 1 lime, sliced into 8

  White Chocolate Mousse Whipped Cream:

- 8 fluid ounces heavy cream
- 3 tablespoons powdered sugar
- ¼ teaspoon pure vanilla extract
- ½ tablespoon white chocolate mousse instant mix

Directions:

1. Preheat the oven to 350F while brushing the graham cracker crust with the egg white. Cover the crust entirely before putting it in the oven to bake for 5 minutes.

2. Whip the egg yolk and condensed milk until they are blended entirely. Add the lime juice then zest to the combination and remain whipping until the mixture is smooth.

3. If you haven't yet, remove the crust from the oven and let it cool. When the crust has cooled, add in the egg combination and bake at 250F for 25 to 30 minutes.

4. When the pie is cooked, put it on a cooling rack to cool. Then place it in the fridge for at least two hours.

5. While waiting for the pie to cool, beat the first three whipped cream ingredients for two minutes (if using a hand mixer). When the mixture is smooth, add in the chocolate mousse and beat to stiff peaks.

6. Remove the pie from the refrigerator, slice it into eight pieces, and garnish each with the white chocolate mousse whipped cream and a slice of lime. Serve.

Nutrition: Calories 500, Total Fat 9 g, Carbs 26 g, Protein 1 g, Sodium 110 mg

BEVERAGE RECIPES

Copycat Starbucks Hibiscus Refresher

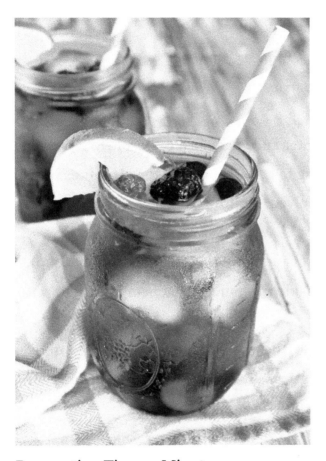

Preparation Time: 5 Minutes

Cooking Time: 5 Minutes

Servings: 2

Ingredients:

- 1 cup of sugar
- 1 cup of water
- 1 green tea bag
- 1 hibiscus tea bag
- 2 cups of water
- 1/4 cup of white grape juice
- 2 tablespoons of simple syrup
- 1/4 cup frozen berries

Directions:

1. Combine the water and sugar in a casserole to create an easy syrup. Bring to a boil then cook for 2 minutes or till the sugar is dissolved. Remove from heat and cool earlier than use.

2. Use the 2 cups of water to brew the inexperienced and hibiscus tea. Enable five mins to steep and then allow to chill down.

3. Pour in a bottle the cooled tea, natural refrigerated syrup, and white grape juice. Shake to blend. Top with a choice of frozen berries and ice.

Nutrition: Calories: 90 Total Fat: 3.5g Saturated Fat: 2g Trans Fat: 0g Cholesterol: 10mg Sodium: 160mg Total Carbohydrates: 11g Dietary Fibers: 1g Sugars: 2g Protein: 4g

Copycat Olive Garden Peach Iced Tea Recipe

Preparation Time: 5 Minutes

Cooking Time: 5 Minutes

Servings: 1

Ingredients:

- 1 cup of sugar
- 1 cup of water
- 2-3 freshly cut peaches
- 3 tea bags
- 6 cups of water

Directions:

1. Put the water, sugar, and peaches in a saucepan over medium heat until they arrive at a boil. Reduce warmth to medium.
2. Crush the peach slices while stirring to dissolve the sugar. As soon because the sugar has dissolved, transfer off the burner, cowl it, and let it rest for about 30 minutes.
3. Brew tea
4. Let water to a boil, then turn it off and permit the tea baggage steep for five minutes.

5. Remove the tea luggage, let them cool to room temperature, then upload syrup to the tea and put it within the refrigerator.

6. Serve on ice and garnish with peach slices as desired.

Nutrition: Calories: 110, Total Fat: 6g, Total Carbohydrate: 34g, Protein: 6g

Passion Fruit Lemonade Starbucks Style

Preparation Time: 10 Minutes

Cooking Time: 5 Minutes

Servings: 2

Ingredients:

- 2 teabags of Tazo Passion iced tea
- 4 cups of water
- 4 cups of lemonade

Directions:

1. Heat the water to the boiling point.
2. Pour the water in a massive jug over the tea bags.
3. Let the tea luggage steep for 10 mins.
4. Remove the tea luggage.
5. Add the lemonade and let it cool in the fridge.

Nutrition: Calories: 119kcal Carbohydrates: 29 g Protein: 0 g
Fat: 0 g Saturated fat: 0 g Cholesterol: 0 mg Sodium: 27 mg
Sugar: 27 g Calcium: 8 mg

Copycat Chick-fil-A Frosted Lemonade

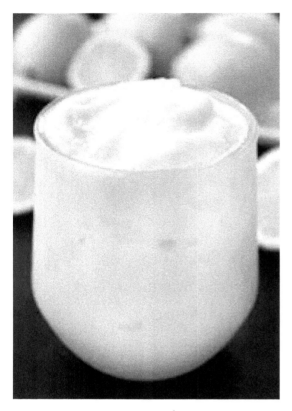

Preparation Time: 5 Minutes

Cooking Time: 0 Minutes

Servings: 4

Ingredients:

- 4 cups of vanilla ice cream
- 1 can of frozen lemonade concentrate
- 1 teaspoon of lemon peel (from 1 lemon)

Directions:

1. Stir all ingredients in a blender till smooth.

2. Fill evenly into 4 glasses and serve immediately.

Nutrition: Calories: 604kcal Carbohydrate: 77 g Protein: 9 g Fat: 29 g Saturated fat: 17 g Cholesterol: 116 mg Sodium: 213 mg Potassium: 525 mg Fiber: 1 g Sugar: 69 g

Starbucks Horchata Frappuccino

Preparation Time: 5 Minutes

Cooking Time: 5 Minutes

Servings: 1

Ingredients:

- 1 cup of water
- 1 cup of brown sugar
- 1 teaspoon of cinnamon
- 1 cup of almond milk
- You can only use 1 cup of vanilla ice cream
- 3-4 tablespoons of cinnamon dolce syrup
- 2 tablespoons of whipped cream
- 1/4 teaspoon of cinnamon

Directions:

1. In a small pan, mix brown sugar and cinnamon.
2. Add the water and let it cook for five mins or till the again of a spoon is full.
3. Allow the airtight container to chill and store.
4. Blend all substances in a blender. Disable it smoothly.
5. Sprinkle with cinnamon and whipped cream as needed.

Nutrition: Calories: 494kcal Carbohydrates: 77 g Protein: 6 g Fat: 19 g

Saturated fat: 10 g Cholesterol: 64 mg Sodium: 466 mg
Potassium: 300 mg Fiber: 1 g Sugar: 72 g

Screaming Zombie

Preparation Time: 5 Minutes

Cooking Time: 5 Minutes

Servings: 1

Ingredients:

- 4 ounces of lemon juice
- 1 tablespoon of sugar
- 3 ounces of orange juice
- 1-ounce light rum
- 1/2 oz Myers Dark Rum
- 1/2-ounce Bacardi Select Rum
- ½ ounce of grenadine

Directions:

1. In a pot, pour the lemon juice and sugar and blend properly.
2. In the equal bowl (or cup) add orange juice and 1 oz. Rum.
3. Half fill with ice a 16-ounce container and pour over it.
4. Let the final three ingredients swim with a spoon in sequence.

Nutrition: Calories: 252, Carbohydrates: 33g, Protein: 11g, Fat: 7g, Saturated Fat: 2g, Cholesterol: 167mg, Sodium: 471mg, Potassium: 171mg, Fiber: 1g, Sugar: 8g

Olive Garden Berry Sangria

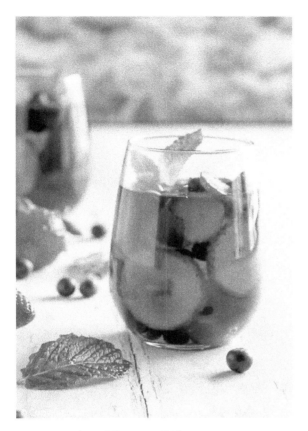

Preparation Time: 5 Minutes

Cooking Time: 0 Minutes

Servings: 8

Ingredients:

- 1 cup of raspberries
- 1 cup blackberries
- Halve 1 cup or a third of strawberries
- 1 cup of sweet wormwood

- 1 cup of grenadine
- 2 cups of raspberry and cranberry juice
- 1.5-liter bottle of Riunite Lambrusco
- 1/2 cup strawberry or cranberry vodka - Optional

Directions:

1. Place berries in the backside of a big gallon jug or two smaller two-quarter jugs.
2. Pour juice, wormwood, and grenadine over berries. Stir to combine.
3. Pour the Lambrusco over the juice-berry combination.
4. Add vodka in case you use to make a more potent drink.
5. Stir to combine.
6. Chill geared up to serve or put together with all pre-chilled substances.
7. Serve with berries in wine glasses.

Nutrition: Calories 303, Total fat 25 g, Saturated fat 11 g, Carbs 4 g, Sugar 1 g, Fibers 0 g, Protein 20 g, Sodium 749 mg

Fireside Coffee

Preparation Time: 5 Minutes

Cooking Time: 0 Minutes

Servings: 4

Ingredients:

- 2 cups of coffee mate
- 1 1/2 cups of instant coffee
- 1 1/2 cups of the instant chocolate mix like Nestle's or Hershey's
- 1 cup of sugar
- 2 teaspoons of cinnamon
- 1/2 teaspoon of nutmeg

Directions:

1. Blend all the substances.
2. Place into 1 cup of warm water 2 heaping teaspoons full of combination.

Nutrition: Calories: 1094kcal Carbohydrate: 198 g Protein: 10 g
Fat: 30 g Saturated fat: 19 g Cholesterol: 89 mg Sodium: 297 mg
Potassium: 921 mg Fiber: 5 g Sugar: 179 g

Copycat Olive Garden Berry Sangria

Preparation Time: 5 Minutes

Cooking Time: 25 Minutes

Servings: 8

Ingredients:

- I used 750 ml red wine Merlot
- 2 cups of cranberry juice
- 1/4 cups of simple sugar syrup
- fresh berries such as strawberries

Directions:

1. Mix all components except the sparkling culmination in a huge container.
2. Stir nicely to combine.
3. Let the mixture relax for some hours before serving.
4. To serve, placing ice in a glass, then clean fruit and sangria, and garnish the glass with a strawberry.

Nutrition: Calories: 147kcal Carbohydrates: 20 g Protein: 0 g Fat: 0 g

Saturated fat: 0 g Cholesterol: 0 mg Sodium: 11 mg Potassium: 162 mg

Fiber: 0 g Sugar: 16 g

CONCLUSION

On that sweet note, we have come to the end of this book. I hope you found the recipes that you were looking for and are raring to get started.

Copycat Recipes are a fun way to play with your food and can help you save money.

How can you save money? For starters, you can find recipes for food that you already have in your kitchen. You'll also save money by purchasing less expensive ingredients. In addition, you can eat leftovers from the night before (which is one of my favorite pastimes). Once you have a list of recipes you want to make, you can sort them out by the type of dish they are. This will allow you to pick and choose dishes that work best for your family, whether it be a quick weekday dinner or a nice Sunday lunch.

After you've chosen the recipes that work best for your family, you'll want to gather the ingredients and equipment needed. Don't forget to take into account the size of your family. If you have a family of 5, it's going to take a bit more food than 2 people.

Also remember that if you are going to make the same dish for your entire family, it will save time and money if you cook once and serve multiple times. This is just a reminder that everything in moderation. Last, but not least, have fun! I hope you enjoy the recipes that you make and that you share them with your friends and family.

I would like to thank all of the wonderful people who helped me with this book. A special thanks to my mom, for helping me find recipes as well as editing my work.

Forget about waiting in line to order food, paying a service tax to your food delivery app, worrying about unhygienic food practices in restaurants, or paying hefty sums for takeout.

You can make these dishes healthier by opting for organic produce. Most restaurants use frozen meats, which are not the best option. You can use fresh meat, seafood, fruit, and vegetables for better results. So, cooking these dishes at home ensures you don't just get the best of taste, but you're even eating healthy food—a total win-win if you ask me. I hope you'll enjoy cooking the dishes in this book. If you have any suggestions, I'd be glad to hear them. Keep in mind that you don't need to own a restaurant to cook restaurant-quality food. In fact, the best restaurants in the world are made on your own stove!

Thank you once again for choosing this book. I wish you luck with your cooking adventures.

CPSIA information can be obtained
at www.ICGtesting.com
Printed in the USA
BVHW051334110421
604614BV00018B/85